My Body Breakthrough

The Unfair Advantage to Getting Your Best Body

Davis Oliver

My Body Breakthrough

Printed by:
CreateSpace Independent
Publishing Platform

Copyright © 2017, Davis Oliver

Published in the United States of America

Book ID: 170130-0068.1

ISBN-13: 978-1546474531
ISBN-10: 1546474536

For more information on 90-Minute Books including finding out how you
can publish your own book, visit 90minutebooks.com or call (863) 318-0464

Here's What's Inside...

Dedications:

Dad- Thanks for inspiring me to write about my transformation and create something great from it. It's because of you this is happening.

Mom- Thanks for reading my book over and over again, you told more people about the book than me. Also, thanks for giving me as many life lessons as the entire book of Proverbs.

Drake- Thanks for giving me constant support and always pushing me. Your own transformation inspires me each day, keep up the hard work.

Coach Harris-Thanks for waking up and pushing me as a person every day to get better in and out of the gym. I dedicate much of my transformation to you, also congrats on your own transformation.

Coleman- As my roommate, thanks for putting up with my lifestyle day after day, you were a big support and have been an amazing friend throughout this entire process.

Last but not least thanks to all my family, friends, Christ School and mentors who have helped support me.

My Body Breakthrough!

When I first started this journey of changing my overall body and health, I didn't know where to start. I was going to bed at one in the morning and eating junk food without thinking about the negative impact it would have on my body. I would feel tired in my high school classes and not even want to go to basketball or football practice. I was getting by in school but really not tapping into my full potential. I knew I wanted a change, but I was confused about where to begin. I had an intense desire to improve my body. I just needed the best plan to attack this goal.

Does this sound like you?

I figured that the best way to change was to lose weight and get ripped, but I didn't know the best ways to do those things. When I first started, I would just eat salads for lunch and dinner and a protein shake for breakfast. I figured the greater a caloric deficit I had, the faster I would lose weight, which was true—I did lose weight, but I lost a lot of weight very quickly.

I would lift weights without knowing if I was really doing the best workout to gain muscle. I wondered if the workout I saw someone else doing was actually right for me. Through extensive research and consulting top advisers to professional body builders in the health and nutrition industry, I learned there is a specific way to lose or gain weight and unique techniques to gain muscle. I want to save you the time and energy of having to research and find the best formula to lose or gain weight, as well as the quickest way to add muscle. I want to give you the easiest way to do what I have done without having to waste a lot of extra time and trouble to get your best body breakthrough.

I have helped guide several people on their journey, but the person I've helped the most is myself. For my best body breakthrough, I learned that the key is discipline and proper diet with the correct workout routine. Once I made this change to my body, people would ask:

- "How did you do it?"

- "What is your diet?"

- "How often do you work out?"

- "Could you make me a diet plan?"

- "Could you create a workout for me to gain size?"

- "You lost all that weight, that quickly; how can I do the same?"

I would answer all of their questions. First, I would make them a proper diet plan based on a few easily answered questions. Then I gave them the recommended macronutrients for their goal of muscle gain or fat loss. The people I have helped either lost their desired weight or are putting on their desired size.

My friend Chad wanted to lose about 20 pounds for college football. He lost about 25 and now has signed on to play Division 1 ("D1") college football. Chad was a typical high school kid who just wanted to lose a few pounds to look better and feel better, and he actually lost the weight, which led to his ability to play football at the next level. Other people have told me that they either lost weight or gained size and they feel much better, both physically and mentally. I have also helped a highly talented high school basketball player named Damon, who will play at the D1 level. Damon wanted to gain size, so I gave him a workout routine and a diet plan for his best body breakthrough, and his results are excellent. In just two months, he has already gained about four pounds. The customized lifting programs I gave to each of them led to them sharing with me something amazing—within just one month, they could see results. The progression in the amount of weight they could lift was exponentially increasing.

My hope is this book educates and inspires you to realize that many others are in your shoes. If you feel you haven't reached your greatest health potential, I am here to tell you that **now** is the time to be the healthiest and fittest you can be.

All it takes is a mindset change and discipline of routine, diet, and workout. It can be done. If you work smart, not just hard (as you do in all other high school achievements like schoolwork, a job, friends, and service), you can have your own best body breakthrough.

You can't control every factor of everything that is important. I am here to tell you that by changing your body and becoming fit, the amount of smart work and discipline is all you have to control. The results will show because no one can alter the outcome or take away your hard work. Many things in high school can consume our time: three hours of homework after school and sports, standardized tests, community service, a job, etc. You don't have complete control over these things to get the results you want - I have been through this process. If you are looking for results you can control, then My Body Breakthrough is for you.

If you stick with a customized plan for quicker and easier results, then the benefits will come.

I was overweight with a good life, but in order for my life to feel great, it just started with a change of mindset to experiencing my own best body breakthrough, and you can too.

To Your Success!

Enjoy this book!

Davis Oliver

Why Most High Schoolers Aren't in the Best Shape of Their Life

Most likely, the problem is that you are a lot like me; you are enjoying moving through high school, making good grades, and having an okay time. But in the back of your mind, you feel that you are missing something. My reason was that I was overweight, and as a result, I wasn't the best version of me that I could be.

I was going to bed at 1:00 a.m. and eating fast food and junk food without thinking about the future repercussions on my body. I would feel tired in class and not really want to go to basketball or football practice. I was going through the motions of high school, just getting by, but really not tapping into my full potential. I have learned that it is nothing to be upset about; it just takes a change of mindset to make a change in your life. I learned that having the right mindset is key to having my best physical body.

Now I look at obstacles in life as hidden opportunities. Being either overweight or underweight is a problem because in everyday life, we each focus our attention on things that hold our time hostage: homework, standardized test preparation, college applications, sports, and clubs. Physicality positions us to achieve greater results.

Focusing on my physical health as a priority enabled me to excel at accomplishing greater results in all areas of my life, the things that have the greatest meaning: faith, family, and friends.

It is not that we are incapable but more that we don't find health and fitness as important as other things and responsibilities. These tend to consume us, leaving little time to focus on physical fitness. But I found the physical fitness success formula to fix this problem. I have been where many of you are, and all it takes is a change in mindset to have a physical transformation. You can learn from all of my countless hours of researching the right diet and macronutrients per body type, to the most effective exercises, these insights will provide you with the quickest and easiest way to your best body breakthrough.

I learned the hard way about the major importance of having a tailored training plan. This will save you time and energy so you will see optimal results without the hassles of the learning curve and lost time that I encountered. I wish I had known all of these things when I first started my journey.

First: Change Your Mindset

In mid-January of 2016, my mindset did a sudden "flip", a sudden change, which then changed my actions. I started working out, taking my diet seriously, and making healthy changes. In eight months, I lost a total of 51 pounds. I went from weighing 210 pounds—down to 159 pounds. I went from being very sick with a gut to very fit, accomplishing six-pack abs. If you are sitting at home reading this, if you want to lose weight and you are overweight, I'm proof that it can be done.

Most people think that losing 51 pounds in that time period is impossible; I'm here to tell you that it's not. In my junior year, when I went to my doctor for a physical (the last time he had seen me was the previous year), he saw that I had lost more than 50 pounds. He shared with me a really interesting fact that just proves how tremendous it is for someone to go through this transformation and how it can severely affect them.

He said, "The two hardest things to do in the medical world are (1) quit smoking, and (2) lose more than 20 pounds. If you make the transformation, it's something to be proud of." It can be done. You hear about people quitting smoking. You hear about people losing weight. You know it can be done; just believe it can happen to you too.

Let me just share a little fact with you about the severity of obesity. In today's world, 74% of people are obese, and 60% of kids from ages 10 to 17 are obese. I won't go into all of the reasons so many people are obese today because there are numerous contributing factors, but I assume that either you're reading this book to become lean and lose weight, or maybe you're wondering what is going into your body that's caused you to become overweight.

The turning point in my case study was making the decision to engage in change for myself. A mentor taught me that all progress begins with the truth. My truth was that my physical shape was not where I wanted to be or where it believed it could be. My mental decision to change allowed me to embrace a process that helped me realize just how much better I could feel and find that thing I was missing. It was the first time I could see my abs, the first time I could break a twenty-minute 5k, the first time I could do more than 10 pull-ups, the first time I had increased energy in class, and the first time I woke up with pure energy. The reason I share my story is I want others to have the same experience. I have been in exactly the same position as many of you are right now, and I have a passion to share what it takes for others like me to experience your best body breakthrough.

The Diet: IIFYM (If It Fits Your Macros)

After mindset, the most important factor in getting the body you want is your diet. There are a lot of different approaches to dieting, so I will share what worked for me. Your diet experience may differ. In fact, I think you should experiment with what works best for you.

My diet mantra is "If It Fits Your Macros",. When I first heard about this diet I did plenty of research. I reviewed information on line and talked to people about it. It sounded too good to be true. Basically, the idea is that you can eat whatever you want if it fits into your macronutrients. Your macronutrients are your fat, proteins, and carbs.

Basically, your body uses fats for energy, growth, and fuel. It's the same with your carbs—it's a fuel energy source. Protein is for your muscle growth, and for your ability to recover from the muscle you're breaking down by lifting, or whatever physical activity you're doing.

Most people are obese because they don't have the right ratios of those macronutrients, so they will eat a lot of high-fat or high-carbohydrate foods or fast food items, which create an insulin spike, especially with the carbs. Your body either uses carbohydrates to replenish muscle glycogen or there's so much of an insulin spike that the excess insulin creates fat.

In the same way, eating excess fats creates body fat in the long term, whereas if you were lifting and eating the right amount of carbs for your activity level, the excess amounts would go to muscle growth instead of fat.

Some of the best ratios for fat loss are about 40% protein, 40% carbs, and 20% fat. These are just suggested amounts. Everyone is different and the macros are very personalized because not everyone reacts in the same way to fats or to carbs. To track your macronutrients, I would suggest that you track the food in grams, to be very specific. The more detailed you are and the more time you put into your diet, the better results you will see.

A caloric deficit means that someone eats fewer than the suggested number of calories in order to lose weight. They would want to eat a certain number of calories fewer than their normal amount of maintenance calories, meaning if they did nothing all day and were idle all day. For example, if they ate about 2,800 calories, they would neither gain nor lose weight. If they wanted to lose weight, they would have to eat in a caloric deficit – that day, they would eat about 500 calories fewer than 2,800 (or 2,300 calories). after a week, for example, you would have about a 3,500-calorie deficit (7 days x 500=3500); so you would lose about a pound because that amount of calories equals a pound.

It all depends on your goals. If you're also trying to bulk up or gain weight, you'd eat about 3,300 calories a day, 500 above the normal 2,800 count. Currently, since I am trying to grow muscle, the ratios are about 180 grams of proteins, 360 grams of carbs, and then 115 grams of fat, but you're not eating crazy unhealthy things.

Many people think this means you can just eat whatever you want. While that's partially true, it's all in moderation. Say it's dinnertime, and you want a slice of pizza, but your grams of fat for that day are already at 66. For you to lose weight, your fat goal is 70 grams for the day (for your needed calories) and your protein grams are low. You need to reach 165 grams of protein for your body weight and size, and you've only had 125 grams. Instead of pizza (although you could eat it at an early point in the day with fat and other carbs to spare), at this point you probably should have chicken or some type of lean protein because that would fit more into your macronutrients.

In another instance, say you're craving a doughnut for breakfast but you haven't had anything to eat. You can have that doughnut, as long as you don't eat more than the rest of your calories for the day. Doughnuts are high in fat and carbs, so just make sure that throughout the rest of the day, you eat items lean in protein that aren't high in carbs, but just fitting your macronutrient goal numbers.

When I first started, I did it all wrong. I cut my calories completely, I tried to eat as little as possible—eating just salads—and then work as hard as I could in the gym, but really I was just hurting my body more than helping it. Once I found my macronutrient calculations (IIFYM), I started seeing immediate improvements.

It was a big breakthrough to find a lean meat option with each meal. You could eat a slice of pizza and doughnut if you wanted, but dieting means you're in a caloric deficit and you get hungry, so you don't really want small portions of things. You've got to have something larger, so you find those things like pancakes, French toast, or waffles, because they are not the worst items for you. You can fit 40 or 50 grams of carbs in your diet, but then realize that you don't need the excess carbs from syrup. Regular syrup is 200 calories per serving. If you substitute sugar-free syrup instead, it tastes very similar, and it's only 15 to 20 calories per the same size serving—about 1/4 of a cup. Part of my success was due to finding out these little things that added up and contributed to early improvements.

Another area where people struggle is in drinking their calories: soda, for example. Coke has about 240 calories, and is pure sugar and carbs. Diet soda is also an option, but is it the best option for you? Probably not but, if you're craving these things it's because you're in a caloric deficit, diet soda is a good option because it will have zero calories, but it's high in sodium. Now there is a Diet Pepsi free of aspartame, it's free from things that could possibly hurt you in the long run, hurt your brain or whatever the scientific establishment suggests.

Another thing that helped me was finding my carb source, so my diet was low in carbs. Vegetables and salads are great options, and also the light or healthier options of foods such as light bread. Instead of 120 calories per slice, light bread has 60 calories per slice with about half the carbs. These may might not taste as great, but in the long run, it's a substitution that will help you feel better and look better, and all you're missing is a very little bit of the taste.

I get asked this question all the time: "Should I lose weight and then bulk up, or can I do both at the same time?" My metabolism has always been a little bit slow, so my amount of protein or calories has been right around 3,200 calories. It's what I eat every day. I track everything that I eat. I've gained weight through this process.

For bulking, you don't want to gain a great excess amount of weight if you still want to have an aesthetic appeal and look good, especially after losing all that weight, or for a hard gainer (someone who has always been very skinny who wants to gain weight). You don't want to gain only a large amount of excess fat. You want to eat the right amount of calories to build muscle and gain a little bit of fat throughout time. That way you're not just becoming fat again. Especially when you first start lifting and implementing the diet, you'll gain muscle mass because it's the first time your muscles have gotten used to this change in diet and exercise.

If you want to lose weight, to see your best results of muscle growth and definition then you will have to start bulking up after you lose the weight (once you use the body breakthrough concept in the right way) because your body will take and use those calories. Once you know how to lose the weight and then add the bulking idea of taking in excess nutrients and using them correctly for your body type, you will still see even better results with added muscle.

Technically, you can lose weight and gain muscle at once if you are losing weight for the first time and then doing some lifting for the first time. You will grow with muscle and lose weight. That's a very rare scenario, and mainly for new people just getting into lifting. If you're overweight, and you've been lifting for a while, your body has already gotten used to stress on its muscles, so you have to lose the weight and then gain it back through bulking—if you want to see results.

For tracking your macros, MyFitnessPal is the main app used by most people in the industry. It's free, though you can buy a more advanced version. I've used the free version for a couple of years now, and it's been fine.

Workout Routine

When I first started going to the gym and working out for sports, I would lift and try all sorts of things, I wouldn't really see the results of lifting, looking better, feeling better, this just wasn't happening. I was doing the motions without seeing the results.

My motivation of change was due to being sick and tired of not being the best me I could be by putting in the work. Change happened when I intensified what I was doing in the gym and really started to take my diet more seriously. I was eating a higher protein diet, less fat, fewer carbs, healthier options, and tracking my macronutrient calories.

I had to do something different in the gym to make this transformation. It started when I set a goal of working out twice a day, not just once a day. I would do cardio and abs in the morning, and lift. Then I would do cardio and abs in the afternoon, and this is how I started to transform.

For the first workout, I'd wake at about 4:30 a.m. and drive with my football coach to the gym. This was a great advantage to have, especially being at an all-boys boarding school, being close with your mentors. Then I would start working out at about 5:15 a.m. I would run for three miles with my elevation mask on. At the beginning, those three miles took me about 26 to 27 minutes;

within six months, I got down to 19 minutes and 15 seconds.

So this is what an elevation mask does. When you put it on, it looks like something Bane would wear (from the Batman movie *The Dark Knight Rises*) and it has different elevation modes. The elevation level modes start at 3,000 feet and goes up to 18,000 feet. You breathe into it and the higher the elevation, the harder it is to breathe. It just works on how fast you're breathing and controlling your breath. It forces you to control your breathing which makes the work harder, but it also helps increase your lung capacity while you're running. Although the elevation mask helps, the real key for improvement is waking up and running every day, increasing your time, pushing yourself each day. When I started doing that, the weight started to melt off, as did the minutes while I ran. Then I would do an ab routine for about 30 minutes in the morning, and then head back to get ready for school.

In my afternoon workout, I would stretch for about 15 minutes, then lift for an hour, then do 30 minutes of ab work; lastly, there was 15 to 20 minutes of some form of cardio, whether it was jumping rope or running hills. I think the huge key for quick fat loss is being at a caloric deficit, by tracking and knowing what I'm eating, how many calories I burned every day, and even recording my exercise. I could tell by how many calories I was in a caloric deficit, which the greater the caloric deficit for that week the more pounds were lost by the end of that week.

There are different apps that you can use on your phone: MyFitnessPal, LoseIt, etc. (I actually played with both of them.) Just open the app and plug in what exercise you did, say 30 minutes of running. Open the app, plug that in, and it will tell you, on average, the pace you're running at. On the treadmill, you can see your pace at a seven or eight-minute mile, or whatever it is. Once you plug in the numbers, it shows approximately how many calories you burnt for the time you did at that pace. Depending on what it is, the amount gets averaged. Say you did 30 minutes of running or a hard ab workout. You could track that on all these things.

You can also use the app for your food, whether you're eating out or making something. After typing in the amount, you get a rough estimate of calories for the item. Not everything will be exact but there will be a close enough estimate; you'll see if you're in a caloric deficit or not. It can be a little bit time-consuming at first, but once you get it set up it's easy to use. There are different solutions for tracking calories, and tracking the amount you work out isn't the best weight loss scenario for everyone. Not everyone wants to put in all of that effort and time, and there are also different scenarios to try such as meal plans or just eating less in portion sizes.

You wouldn't think that, when I started losing weight (when I was lifting), there would be an increase in weight. If you're less than what you weighed you wouldn't think your strength would go up. But by losing the weight, my squat max increased 25 pounds and my clean max increased 40 pounds. Some things stayed the same but overall, my strength improved just from losing weight. People think they're going to lose their strength when they lose the weight, but that's not true. They'll feel better and stronger. When you're losing that weight, you're using a lot of energy. It takes a lot of energy to hold that kind of weight, and you're not putting your real energy into the things that you could be doing. When you lose that weight, it allows you to put more energy into growing muscle mass instead of having to burn off fat.

What My Workout Looks Like Now and what I Recommend for Others

"What does your workout look like now?" That was a common question I got after losing weight. The workout routine for me was to look more muscular. The aesthetic part of it is different for everyone because it depends on your goals, whether you want to be more aesthetic, gain more strength, run a marathon, etc. I found that my goal of losing weight is what most people consider bodybuilding or hypertrophy training (weight lifting), which doesn't place the focus on the weight as much as the form and isolating the muscle you're trying to use and grow.

Over time, I've learned and gained from others' routines for muscle growth, and found the best routines that work for me. There are very detailed programs for six-day splits, which means about one muscle group per day, and then one rest day. Then I help individuals with My Body Breakthrough by making a routine for the individual. I help people start from the ground up by giving them set days of different exercises for either a four or a six-day split. I usually recommend a four-day split plan for beginners, which is very easy to transfer into a six-day plan.

With each specific exercise, we focus on the form and the time that muscles are in tension. Whatever the exercise is, there should be a solid squeeze or a hold for each rep with this muscle; that's how I train. Then I will give a rep number that I learned and noticed is best for each muscle group, and that muscle alone. One of the key things that does impact muscle growth is knowing how to hit the muscle from different angles properly.

Lastly, after a while with the same program, the muscle gets used to the routine. When you feel you have reached a mature level and maximum growth with that program, we will start a new program. Whether it's to build up a better overall foundation or to work on weak points, I found that hypertrophy training leads to the best overall shredded and lean, bulked muscle definition for the aesthetic physique. This is the technique many physique and body builders recommend and use today.

Goals

High school is a crazy, hectic time with grades, sports, family, testing, service, friends, etc. How do you create a happy balance of all these things? Setting goals was the second way I used to balance all these obstacles. Many people travel through life following a routine they adapt to, but a high school routine can get more and more hectic, whether the homework load is increasing, AP testing is near, family issues or commitments arise, etc.

What seemed to be an easy and not-so-bad routine all of a sudden can become strenuous and challenging. This was the case for me until I saw that if I set goals, all of the pop-ups events that take place in high school can be balanced.

This is how to do it. On Sunday night, before I go to bed, I step back and think about what I have planned for tomorrow while reviewing my school calendar. On a sticky note app on my computer, I type out what I will finish by that day, whether it's my math homework for the week by Tuesday night, or to wake up during the week at 4:30 a.m. just to have that goal set to work out.

By setting a goal, and typing or writing it out, I know I will get it done It is imperative to write it down in order for it to happen by setting written goals, you can cope with what seems to be just too much. Also, goals can be set as something to reach over longer periods of time, not just as reminders or a schedule. It doesn't matter how crazy the goal is, whether it's to lose 50 pounds in the next eight months, get a 4.0 GPA, run a five-minute mile, or get into an Ivy League college.

Whether your goal is big or small, by writing it down or just visualizing it, when you finally reach the goal or the date you set for the goal, you can look back and see what you have achieved. If you don't reach the goal, you can see how far you've come. Keeping constant goals in life can help you.

When you feel like giving in, trust me, we've all been there. When you get done with school, you remember the hard work you've done, but you also recognize how far you've come from where you were. What you have achieved helps you realize you can do it, you can balance high school stress and get through to achieve greatness. Too many times in high school, teachers and parents (and even our fellow classmates) remind us of what we have done wrong, but if you look back and remember what goals you have achieved or nearly reached, we can see how far we have come. It's okay, even beneficial, to look back and admire the past, but take what you have learned and gained in the past and apply it towards your future growth.

Having a goal to aim at is a necessary step to becoming what you want to see. Older people love to ask me, "What are your goals in five or ten years down the road?" I think the best question is, "What is your health goal in the next year?" A lot of people think in the long term, but they don't think about the short-term to medium-term with their health. When you are dieting, it's easy to stray away from a goal, especially the way you want to see your body, because it's hard to stay on track when you don't see immediate results.

When I first started dieting, I really just wanted to lose about 15 pounds, but then I lost that 15 pounds and I said, "No, my goal is a six-pack—whatever weight I have to do to get to a six-pack." I did that, but it was sloppy. I cut my calories too low, starved myself sometimes, and lost some hard-earned muscle mass. I'd be grumpy during the day because I was always hungry.

By setting goals with If It Fits Your Macros model, and slowly reaching them by being patient, you'll gradually see the results and stay with it longer because you know you will get to these set goals without hurting your daily life along the way.

Sometimes, when you're dieting, you'll feel a craving, like, "Oh, I need this." You will have these setbacks. We're all human. We make the mistakes that set us back, but it's our recovery that matters. One doughnut that week will not kill you as long as you stick with the program in the long run and set that desired goal. In weight loss, it's not about that one instant of eating something you were sorry about. It's about the average throughout the week. Say you mess up that one time during the week; it's the multiple weeks adding up that lead to the total fat loss because weight loss is a long-term thing.

The more detailed attention you pay to your diet, the better results you'll see, but if you mess up, it's not the end of the world. Just keep the end goal in mind and realize when you mess up, that you can recover by eating fewer calories tomorrow and throughout the day. The key is having that something that sets you up for progress throughout that week.

Why Being F.I.T. (Fun In Training) in High School Makes for a Better Experience

While I was growing up, when I was hungry, I ate what I wanted or whenever I wanted . Not once did I think about what I was putting in my body and how it would affect me or, for that matter, know that it would affect me. It took until my junior year to figure this out. What you put into your body really affects your body more than anything else. When I finally started to lose weight, I just tried to eat healthier: salads, fewer carbs, and fewer fatty fried foods. I lost about 10 pounds over a month, but not once during that month did I look back on the calories or macronutrients, or anything I know now. This was my biggest mistake.

"Why is it a mistake?" you might ask. This mistake was due to a lack of knowledge that would have led to optimum results. As I said earlier, the right ratios of macronutrients lead to more successful weight loss and healthier weight loss without the degradation of muscle.

You're probably wondering, "How does this affect high school?" Well, I've learned about moving from being fat to pretty fit in high school. Now I know what I put into my body will determine what I get out. If I eat and drink a lot before I go to bed, I will weigh more and be bloated in the morning. I also know that eating any kind of sugar makes me feel sick in the morning and makes it harder for me to wake up. After a workout, if I wanted to grow to get optimal results, I needed to refill glycogen levels by eating a certain amount of fat, protein, and a high amount of carbs within an hour for optimal results. You need these nutrients to stay full throughout the workout. The more I figured this out, the better I performed and the more muscle I gained. I would love to share all these secrets with you and the true details on my body breakthrough.

The reason I started to find all these different ways to lose weight and make my body more effective was that I started to see positive results much quicker. Let's be honest, who doesn't want to see results quickly? Results build confidence and encourage us to do more. Who doesn't love to succeed, and become more confident in high school? It improves morale, motivation, grades, weight room gains, and sports performance. Diet improves so much of our daily lives that it's really hard to realize, which is truly something amazing to have in high school if you start early.

We all know that high school can be a little awkward: acne, hormones, etc. If we control something like our health through diet and exercise, we are ahead of the program in life; plus, things like hormones are uncontrollable. Why not control the one thing you can control, i.e. health and fitness through diet? I struggled with all of these things, but one thing that truly built my charisma and confidence was being shredded and eating healthy. Not only is eating a key for confidence in high school, it is also very important for sports performance.

When I first started high school sports, I used my overweight size to my advantage in football and basketball. As I got older and moved up in levels of sports competition, I noticed that my size wasn't enough for success. I was missing key factors like speed, endurance, and strength, which would also help improve my skills. After training and dieting rigorously, I was one of the fastest and strongest kids on the football team, but for basketball, it was too late. My weight had caught up to me; I lost my skills and have given up on the game.

Now, not only am I in good shape, I'm in the kind of shape that means I don't get tired from practice; instead, now I lift and run after practice. I tell you this, not to impress you, but to show the importance of diet and how it can positively affect you in high school. That is why we go to school, right? Also, my grades have improved. I was a pretty good student in my freshman year. I started with a 4.2 in my junior year and finished with a 4.65. During that transformation, you may be thinking that my energy levels went down, but in reality, they didn't. My GPA got better, and I would attain the highest GPA of my high school career to date. It wasn't because I got smarter. I had more of a work ethic, more energy, and more of the ability to go further with my academics.

Since I ate healthier foods, I had more energy to study after school, which reduced the amount of time I needed to study at night; this also allowed me to go to bed earlier, get better rest, and succeed more. To be honest, I can't really think of a scenario that it might hurt in high school to be healthy, happy, and fit. All I have experienced are the positives, not any negatives.

I want to reiterate that in high school, the time of our lives, if we are fat and unhealthy, we truly aren't taking advantage of two important things: 1) our metabolism and 2) our ability to be active. All high school students have plenty of time to go out and be active, but so few rarely do. That's the problem with our generation—we aren't being fit now. More fat kids now just create more fat people later. This is why now about 74% of the US is obese.

I beg you not to become fit just for high school. Do it so you won't hurt yourself in your adult years, when you don't have time to run, climb, lift, etc. Instead, when you get older, you have to do things your parents probably are consumed with now: work, kids, meetings, obligations, etc.

The other important factor is metabolism, or how fast your body burns calories. Whether it's slow or fast for you now, know that when you get older, it gets a whole lot slower. Take advantage of what you can do now and how you can lose weight.

I want to leave you with some pointers about what we put in our body, a reminder it actually matters.

We look better, and are more confident during high school, which can be a less confident time. From sports and studying, starting with our prime years, energy is a good focus to develop now for when your metabolism reduces in later years. Take a stance to become and stay physically fit. Start by asking yourself, how can I get My Best Body Breakthrough?

.

The Devil's Temptation

The Devil's Temptation is different for everyone, but for a lot of us, it means things like doughnuts and pizza. This section is about how to handle the obstacles that interfere with your diet and your training, and the goals you have set in high school.

All of these things are coming from my experience. Going to a boarding school and having a family that loves their fair share of sweets, I know that temptation can be great for unhealthy foods. Remember, I used to be fat. I still crave things. The cravings really never go away. The only thing that changes is how well you deal with them. When dieting, the hardest thing to do about temptations is to avoid them or substitute for them.

Boarding school was hard because of the way they motivated students and tempted us to do well in academics and service by food, from doughnuts for service hours to pizza for keeping our room clean. This is the question you're probably asking yourself: "How do I avoid the temptations?"

It is hard. As a human, I've fallen to temptation. Trust me I know how hard it is to stay on track with dieting. My roommate has the quickest metabolism on the face of the earth, and all he eats is junk food. One way I deal with it is by pure willpower.

If you can keep in your head the goal of what you want to become and why you're dieting, it will truly help you curb the cravings.

Two, there are better alternatives like the list I shared above. There are plenty of healthy alternatives to some of our favorite junk foods, such as desserts. When I was dieting, my favorites were peanut butter FitCrunch bars and cookie dough Quest bars. They taste like their description. The FitCrunch tastes like a peanut butter Snickers, and the Quest bar tastes like chocolate chip cookie dough.

Those are some of my favorite healthy alternatives to fix the quick cravings. There are great options for meals to. I shared this earlier, but for pancakes, substitute sugar-free syrup; if you don't want empty carbs, substitute Kodiak cakes. They are basically made like a typical pancake, but there is added protein instead of just empty carbs, so you do get some added protein.

There are plenty of healthy alternatives listed in this book that I wish someone would have shared with me before I went out and spent money on things that taste like crap. When I was dieting, I always got the question, "Why aren't you hungry? You basically eat nothing." They're partially right. I didn't eat much, but I curbed hunger by finding foods with low calories and large volume. Also, I didn't eat as much in the morning and saved my calories at night for when I was hungrier.

These were the two main strategies that helped me to avoid going to bed hungry.

Another idea is to drink coffee or zero-calorie drinks; even water will help you curb your hunger. In high school, you can't always control what food is made or decide where you go to eat, but nearly every place you go has a somewhat healthy option. I couldn't control what was made in boarding school, but I could control what I decided to eat in the dining hall. Luckily, we had a salad bar for every meal, and they usually had a fairly decent protein option, so it wasn't that hard to stay on track.

Eating out with friends is hard, especially in high school. Many of your friends will tempt you. "Come on, man. Enjoy yourself. Get a burger," or "It's just one time. Just freaking eat." At this point, there have been times where I caved, and that's fine. One time won't destroy your diet or your gain unless you decide to go to Golden Corral and eat the entire buffet. If you decide to break down with a meal, don't let it destroy your ambition or mindset. Maybe do some more cardio that day or just decide that that was a cheat meal, and you will come back tomorrow and hit the gym really hard because you have all those calories to use as energy. Stay on track with your diet when eating out, but if you cave in, know that it's okay to crave but recover from it, because it won't set you back that far.

This topic leads to my next point: cheat meals. One of the first problems of dieting is when people stay on a diet for a long time and never feed their cravings. When they finally get off the diet, they go hog wild and binge eat everything they were craving. That's why I recommend a cheat meal. Depending on how fast you want to lose weight, it can appear once a week or once every two weeks. Cheat meals are necessary for the reason mentioned earlier, but not only for glycogen. It's also to build a mindset of appreciation and make you realize that in the future, you really only want to eat things that are worthwhile in calories. If you don't love something know you can look forward to eating what you really love at the end of the week or two weeks, as your cheat meal. This is the only way I found you can truly stay on track but still enjoy your high school life.

To recap some points from this chapter:

1) How to stay on track with temptations—curbing your hunger strategies;

2) Eating out with friends in high school and sticking with this diet;

3) Knowing how to recover diet mishaps

4) Volume over quality—just staying full, especially when dieting. Remember that the choice is always fuel over taste.

5) Cheat meals—having rewards but moving forward afterwards.

Receiving Advice from Others

High school students think we know a lot, but in reality, there's so much for us to learn. Through my fitness and health journey, I met people who had been in the health and fitness industry for a while, and I have gained an immense amount of knowledge from them. Most recently, I met a 56-year-old trainer out of Miami named Gage. Gage doesn't look a day over 30 years old. He is a physique body builder who was on the cover of *Men's Health*; I gained a lot of information and knowledge from him.

I had the distinct privilege to gain great insight and train with an IFBB (International Federation Body Building) professional classic physique bodybuilder named Steve. He is also an entrepreneur who owns his own company as a competition prep coach and competition posing coach. Both these competitors have been in the industry for over two decades. From them, I learned some of the best advice I've ever been given. Although they are different in age and points in their careers, in different walks of life, both taught me similar things that led to their successes over the years, in and out of the gym. Let me share a few with you.

The first thing I learned was not to let the gym control you. "You control the gym," meaning there is no reason to be in the gym over an hour and 15 minutes, or at least that's what they said. They don't know each other, but they both have the same opinion on time in the gym; each of their workouts lasts between 45 minutes and an hour and 15 minutes.

When I first started, I thought that the longer I was in the gym, the greater results I would see, which was just false. They said that if you spend too much time in the gym, you will over train, which will hurt your body and muscles more than by allowing them time to grow.

Another piece of advice is consistency, which is important for either a diet or time in the gym. When I asked what they ate, Gage told me he ate the same thing every day: whole wheat pancakes, peanut butter, Dave's Bread, and egg whites. Then lean meat, vegetables, and potatoes for lunch and dinner.

For Steve, the pattern was very similar. Every day, he would eat five or six meals of the same thing every day. Very rarely would either of them stray away from the diet, and the same with the gym. They would follow their schedule. Whether they liked their lifting routine or not they stuck with it. Most teenagers find it hard to be consistent with their busy lives, but being able to put your goals above other things that are important in your busy life is the key to success.

A third piece of knowledge was the importance of rest days. Most teenagers are either so hungry for a goal, but don't know how to truly achieve it, or they're so unmotivated, they don't bother to try.

That was not a characteristic of either Steve or Gage. I had thought the harder I worked without rest, the better results I would get, but in muscularity, that is not the case. They both said a rest day was most important for both muscle and mental growth. It allows for time to refill the body with nutrients, repair the body in the upcoming days, and allow muscles to repair and collect nutrients.

In each day spent with them, I learned many meticulous health tips, from lifts to rep count to breathing, all of these things can be learned through the My Body Breakthrough program. I wish I had these invaluable insights when I started my journey. Whether you are trying to lose or gain weight, everyone needs to start somewhere, but starting the right way with the right things will make your transformation that much easier. Through lots of time and research and mistakes, I had to find all of these fitness and health tips that you can now learn to. Take the stress and difficulty out of making your body transformation.

The Mistakes People Make When Trying to Undergo a Body Transformation

First, avoid the biggest mistake I made right off the bat; wanting my goal too much without embracing the need of a system with a process— smarter over harder. I thought the harder I worked while eating less food, the more weight I would lose. True, I lost the weight, but I also lost the muscle. Another mistake was that I thought the more I worked my muscles, the more the muscle would grow, so I wouldn't take any days off. This actually hurt me more than it helped me. My mentors taught me that my muscles were so fatigued they couldn't absorb the glycogen needed to perform muscle synthesis to grow. All of these are very common mistakes, but trust me, resting your body and eating a sufficient number of calories to lose weight (but not muscle) is key. I share all of these details so others can avoid a harder-over-smarter outcome.

Another mistake is focusing way too much on the weight. When lifting, the only thing weight does is test your strength; the amount of weight you lift has nothing to do with how ripped you will look. Instead, the process is about hypertrophy, and the amount of time the muscle is under tension from that weight. Heavier weight is an important factor but don't max out all the time.

The muscles still need to be reasonably pushed to be torn down in order to be built back up, but don't go for maxes to be cool.

How to Have Your Own Body Breakthrough and Get Your Best Body Yet...

The process I've designed is very simple. It starts with a simple sign-up page on our website (**www.MyBodyBreakthrough.com)**. I will then send my simple seven questions to answer. This will help me create a personalized diet plan for you to either increase lean bulk or to lose weight and retain muscle. Based on the selected plan below, further steps will be carried out to individualize each program.

You can also join the free My Body Breakthrough educational vblog for the latest breakthroughs tips and techniques so you can get the greatest results in the shortest amount of time. You can sign up now and get a free gift for joining the My Body Breakthrough community, at **www.MyBodyBreakthrough.com,** an easily downloadable report that tells you the three best things for your body right now.

Visit website **www.MyBodyBreakthrough.com** to get your desired level of support.

Progress Package Programs:

Package One
(A S150.00 Value)

Basic Body Breakthrough:
Three-Month Package

- $29.95

- Customized Nutrition Plan to add or lose desired weight. (Includes a macro intake menu for the quickest results.)

- Supplementation recommendations

- Customized Workout Plan to build foundation or overcome weak point areas.

Package Two (Most Popular)
(A $250.00 Value)

My Body Breakthrough Level One:
Six-Month Package

- $59.95
- Includes copy of book
- Special Body Blog
- Customized Nutrition Plan to add or lose desired weight. Includes macro intake menu for the quickest results.
- Customized Workout Plan to build foundation or overcome weak point areas.
- Supplementation recommendations
- Personal 20-minute monthly progress check-in call.

Package Three
(A $500.00 Value)

The Complete Package
Total Body Breakthrough Complete
Customization Program

My Body Breakthrough Level Two:
12-Month package

- $149.95 annually

- Full email access or text with any questions around nutrition or workout.

- Supplementation recommendations

- Includes copy of book

- Special Body Blog

- Customized Nutrition Plan to add or lose desired weight. (Includes macro intake menu for the quickest results.)

- Customized Workout Plan to build foundation or overcome weak point areas.

- Personal 30-minute monthly progress check-in call

As a bonus for joining, I will send you five of the Top Nutrition Tips (I wish I knew then what I know now) which are specific bullet-point tips that answer specific questions on nutrition. Also, five of The Top Gym Tips (I wish I knew then what I know now) are specific bullet-point tips that answer specific questions in lifting.

If you have questions send me an email: **info@MyBodyBreakthrough.com**.

The best thing to do is to visit www.MyBodyBreakthrough.com and sign up.

Medical Disclaimer

My Body Breakthrough author or support team are not licensed medical professionals. *My Body Breakthrough* strongly recommends that you consult with your physician before beginning any exercise or diet programs.

You should be in good physical condition and be able to participate in all exercise.

My Body Breakthrough is not a licensed medical care provider and represents that it has no expertise in diagnosing, examining, or treating medical conditions of any kind, or in determining the effect of any specific exercise, diet, or meal plans related to medical conditions.

You should understand that when participating in any meal plan, diet or exercise program, there is the possibility of physical injury. If you engage in this meal plan, diet, exercise or exercise program, you agree that you do so at your own risk, are voluntarily participating in these activities, assume all risk of injury to yourself, and agree to release *My Body Breakthrough* and discharge from any and all claims or causes of action, known or unknown, arising out of any *My Body Breakthrough* negligence.

Biography:

I was born in Springfield, Ohio, and raised in Winter Park, Florida through elementary and middle school. The start of high school I moved to Arden, NC with my family to attend Christ School, an all boys' boarding school. It wasn't until late into my junior year that I found the inspiration to make my own body breakthrough transformation, going from 210lbs. to 159lbs. Within eight months I learned a lot about what I did wrong and what I did right during my physical transformation. I am currently 18 years old and finishing my senior year at Christ School. I am looking forward to attending The University of North Carolina at Chapel Hill in the fall of 2017. I went from losing all that weight to gaining a lot of muscle weight back through the My Body Breakthrough lean bulking program. Since that last day of weighing 159lbs., I now weigh a lean 185lbs. a year later. I created The My Body Breakthrough system to save others the time and energy I had to encounter through finding these unfair advantages. Allow me to provide you with insightful direction with an easier and proven process that you can start right now!